One Way Ticket to Florida

One Way Ticket to Florida

~

LOVING SOMEONE WITH ALZHEIMER'S

S.R. Crawley

Scotchwood Hill Publishing Services

This book is dedicated to Darrell Keller, a newfound cousin I connected with, thanks to Facebook. Without his help, this story never would have happened. Thank you for all your help. This book is a tribute to my grandparents. We all long for a love that is willing to do anything for us. A love that reflects our heavenly Father's divine love for us. Never give up hope. This book is a way of sharing this story with my family and future generations.

Contents

Dedication   v

1   Chapter One   1

2   Chapter Two   5

3   Chapter Three   8

4   Chapter Four   12

5   Chapter Five   15

6   Chapter Six   18

7   Chapter Seven   21

8   Chapter Eight   25

9   Chapter Nine   31

10 Chapter Ten   36

11 Chapter Eleven   40

12 Chapter Twelve   44

13 Chapter Thirteen   49

14 Chapter Fourteen   53

15 Epilogue   58

16 Authors Note   60

17 Newspaper Articles   61

18   Photos   64

19   Also by Sherri Croom   68

1

~

Chapter One

Arnvel sat at the kitchen table, loading a .25 caliber pistol. He inserted the last bullet and slid it home. The sensation of hot needles probing every joint sent pain through his hands and up his arm. The warm patches from inflammation itched worse than measles. He laid the pistol down on the table and shuffled to the bathroom. After relieving himself and washing his hands, he opened a bottle of hydrocodone from the medicine cabinet. He had to get his pain under control before his friend arrived to pick him up. He swallowed the pill with a gulp of water from the bathroom sink.

He trudged back towards the kitchen, feeling like he was walking in sludge. Reclaiming the pistol, he decided to wait in the living room. He plopped down on the sofa. His knees were not what they used to be.

Laying the pistol on the coffee table, he pulled one of the throw pillows onto his lap to elevate his hands. Closing his eyes, he replayed the events that led him to this point.

* * *

Arnvel had been an Army medic when he and Irene first met. Early into his career, he developed rheumatoid arthritis and was soon discharged. After the Army, he worked managing movie theaters. When he reached the age of 50, the disfigurement and pain in his hands became worse until he could no longer work.

When Arnvel met Irene, she had three children. He didn't have children, and they had none together, but he treated her kids as his own. All three children passed away in their early forties and late fifties. A person never gets over outliving their children. You deal with it daily. Arnvel and Irene were all that remained in their little family.

The couple exited the doctor's office and started down the long hallway. Irene usually marveled at the beautiful artwork that hung on each side. She said the paintings belonged in an art gallery instead of a doctor's office. Her favorite piece was of the beach. Seagrass bordered a sandy path that led to an ocean. Three seagulls flew above the cresting waves, and a boat sailed toward the horizon. She said the piece reminded her of their life in Florida. Today, she walked past them as if they didn't exist.

Arnvel took her hand. She faced him with a slight grin. Tears streaked down her face. "It will be okay, Irene. I'll be with you every step of the way."

When the doctor said Alzheimer's, Arnvel felt his insides rise, and he swallowed hard. He knew something was wrong but refused to believe it might be Alzheimer's or dementia. There was no denying it now.

He swallowed again to clear the lump in his throat and to hold back the flood behind the dam. He had to keep his emotions together. Irene's sobs broke his trance, and he knew there would be many more, so many more. He watched as her mouth moved, but she couldn't form words. He slid his chair closer, wrapped his arm around her, and gripped her hand. "What do we need to do?" Arnvel asked the doctor.

Arnvel called for a taxi before leaving the doctor's office, and it waited for them when they came out. He had quit driving years ago due to the arthritis in his hands. The taxi company was quite familiar with them because they always initiated a conversation and got to know each driver personally. Irene often baked them cookies, and Arnvel tipped them well. The drivers treated the duo as their adopted grandparents.

When the driver saw them come out, he hurried to open the door for them and helped Irene in. She slid to the other side without saying a word. "Is she all right, Mr. Roberts?" the concerned driver asked. It was apparent something was wrong. They were not the happy, joking couple he had dropped off earlier.

"Nothing we can't handle, Benjamin." Arnvel stepped into the car, retook Irene's hand, and looked straight ahead.

Benjamin leaned down and whispered into Arnvel's ear, "I'm here if you ever want to talk." Then he shuts the car door.

When they got home, Irene went straight to bed. Arnvel tried to get her to eat something, but she said she was too tired to eat. He didn't force the issue. He felt the same way. He sat in his chair with the TV on, paying no attention.

Alzheimer's. The word hammered his brain like the agonizing pounding of a migraine. His lap held the pamphlets the doctor sent home with him. His twisted fingers ached and burned like lava under his skin as he read through them. The more he read, the more scared he became. He couldn't help but wonder how he would handle all that was to come. Would he be able to care for her as her disease progressed? Positioning himself straighter, he thought, *"I was a medic, for goodness sake. I can do this!"*

He put away the pamphlets and looked in on Irene. Entering the room, he found her asleep. He tucked her blanket under her chin and kissed her good night. He crossed the room to his bed and picked up their wedding picture from the dresser. He placed it on his nightstand and tucked himself in. He gazed at the young lovers, arms entwined, and strolled down memory lane until he fell to sleep — the last peaceful night of sleep he was to have.

After Irene's diagnosis, the disease progressed faster. It was easier when he didn't know. They laughed it off when he said, "You would forget your head if it wasn't on your shoulders," or "You gotta run faster to catch that train of thought." They both knew the joke was over, and he was witnessing the symptoms as they happened and dreaded what was to come.

She no longer recalled the names of her neighbors or the day of the week. What broke Arnvel's heart the most was that she often referred to him as Grandpa. The first time this happened, it devastated him. He had seated her at the table and placed a bib around her neck. She looked down at the plate and made a face like a child. "I don't like peas."

"Then eat what you do like, dear." Arnvel took a bite of his. "Mmm, they sure are good, though."

"Grandpa, I'm not hungry. I think I will go to bed." She got up from the table and said, "Good night." She headed toward the bedroom.

His eyes filled with tears as he watched her shuffle away.

2

Chapter Two

The first of many scares happened one beautiful morning, proving terror doesn't only come during the dark and gloomy. The day Arnvel learned the meaning behind the words, "Things can change at the drop of a hat," Irene was still asleep when Arnvel looked in on her. Deciding to drink his morning coffee on the front porch, he let his hands absorb the heat from the mug. He smiled and waved to the neighbors as they left for work. "Good morning!" he yelled. They returned his greetings.

George, from across the street, came over with his coffee. "Good morning, Roberts. Do you mind some company?" George was younger than Arnvel, but both men were military and addressed each other by their last names.

"Morning, Davis, don't mind at all. Have a seat." Arnvel set his coffee mug beside him. Over the years, he had become self-conscious about handling things in front of people. Often, he felt people staring at his disfigurement.

"You're taking advantage of this good morning, I see." He sat beside Arnvel.

"Oh yeah, there aren't many left."

"How is Irene doing? I haven't seen her out in a couple of days."

Arnvel took a deep breath before he tried to speak. Other than the doctors, he had not talked to anyone about her worsening condition. "She's not doing so good. There are days that she doesn't know who I am. I look at her, Davis, and I see the woman I fell in love with, but when I look into those eyes, I see her confusion." The tears fell. "What hurts the most is the fear in her eyes when she can't remember me."

"Roberts, I'm so sorry..." A thud followed by a cry came from behind the house. George flew off the porch, disappearing around the house before Arnvel could get up and off the porch.

As Arnvel came around the corner of the house, he saw George kneeling beside Irene. He was cradling her head and telling her to lie still. Arnvel's heart stopped, and his lungs refused to work. An eternity passed before he got to her. "Oh my God, Irene! Are you all right? What happened?"

Irene held her right arm close to her chest. Arnvel could see blood on her leg, but he couldn't tell where it came from.

"She's all right, Roberts, but she may have broken her arm. She needs to see a doctor.

"I'm all right, Arnvel. I just came out to check on the kids and missed the step. This nice man heard me and came to help."

At the hospital, while they were doing x-rays on Irene, Arnvel tried to fill out the stack of papers they had given him. He failed miserably. His fingers refused to cooperate. Head hung low. He walked back up to the window and asked the lady for help.

"Sure," she said smiling, "We have someone to help with that."

Three hours later, the taxi pulled up in the couple's driveway. Irene's scraped leg was bandaged, and her sprained arm was in a sling. The cab driver helped her while Arnvel unlocked the door.

Mindful of her injuries, Arnvel seated her at the kitchen table. "I'm going to fix us a sandwich. I know you must be as hungry as I am."

"I could eat something now that you mentioned it. Oh, how about a grilled egg and cheese sandwich?"

He hoped to get away with making ham and cheese sandwiches, but she had not expressed this much excitement about food in quite a while.

He would not let his pain stop him from making her happy. "You must have read my mind. Two grilled egg and cheese coming up."

He blundered a couple of times as he prepared their sandwiches, but nothing too serious. Irene watched in silence until cracking an egg became squashing an egg, and she laughed. "Don't laugh at me," he teased, cleaning the mess. He placed both sandwiches on a paper plate and set the plate between them. "They are not pretty, but I don't think even I could ruin the grilled egg and cheese taste."

Her excitement was gone, but she smiled at him as she picked up her sandwich and took a bite. "They are perfect."

Later, during their nightly routine, they tucked themselves into their beds, "Good night, Irene, I'll see you in my dreams."

"Good night, and I'll be there. Did you check on the kids before you came to bed?"

He didn't correct her. "They are safe and sound." He closed his eyes and wept, not only for her but for himself. In her world, their children were still alive. He felt envious.

3

∾

Chapter Three

Irene rocked on the front porch most of the day. Arnvel came out carrying two plastic glasses of iced tea in the crook of his arm. Before Irene's illness, he never attempted to carry two of anything. He had learned to do a lot of things but with consequences.

"Grab these for me, please." He stood in front of her, but she didn't see him. "Irene!" She blinked and stared at him. He could tell she didn't recognize him. He did what every pamphlet told him to do. He called her by name and reminded her of his name. "Irene, it's me, Arnvel."

She crossed her arms and returned to rocking, "I know who you are, silly."

"Well then, will you please get your tea before I drop it and make a mess?"

"Oh, I'm sorry. Let me grab that."

Letting out a grunt, he dropped into his chair and sipped his drink.

She took a drink of her tea and licked her lips. "Mmm, that's good stuff." Still holding her glass, she continued to rock.

He made several attempts to start a conversation, but she either offered a simple reply or nothing at all. He decided to keep silent and let her enjoy whatever memory she was reliving. She had a smile on her face. They continued to rock the afternoon away. He dozed off a few times, but he wasn't sure about her. He didn't catch her napping if she did. He noticed the setting sun and drew her attention to its beauty.

She reached over and took his hand, "Do you know a sunset is God's way of putting a crown on another one of His perfectly planned days?"

He remembered her telling him that on their first date, and he had heard her say it many times since then. "What a beautiful thought, Irene."

They watched the sunset until the sun was completely out of sight. Arnvel's stomach made a grumbling noise.

"Was that your stomach?" Irene laughed.

"No, that was you," he joked. "I guess that's my cue. It's supper time. Do you want to help me fix us a hot dog?"

"No, I don't think so. I'll sit out here for a while longer."

"All right, I'll come to get you when it's ready."

She didn't respond. A couple of chirping birds in a nearby tree had captured her attention. Smiling, he went inside to microwave hot dogs.

When everything was finished, he went to bring her in. "Supper's ready," he yelled as he approached the screen door. She didn't answer, and when he opened the door, she was not on the porch. He looked up and down the street and didn't see her. He called out her name but got no answer. He walked to the back of the house, thinking maybe she was there. She was nowhere in sight. He called 9-1-1.

Within an hour, police officers and concerned neighbors combed the neighborhood looking for Irene. Arnvel stood on the porch, looking in one direction and then in the other, praying he would see Irene walking up the sidewalk. He felt sick with worry. He knew something like this could happen. He had read the warnings about Alzheimer's patients wandering. *How could I have been so stupid?* He suddenly felt hot. His heartbeat was faster. He felt he couldn't get enough air. Instinctively, his hand went to his chest, and he started to breathe faster.

Arnvel felt someone touch his shoulder.

"Mr. Roberts, would you like to go inside where you can be more comfortable?"

"No," he answered between breaths, "I'll wait out here." His vision became blurry, and he realized he was having a panic attack. He had not experienced an attack since the Army. The next thing he knew, he was eased into one of the rocking chairs. Again, he heard the male voice.

"Mr. Roberts, look at me!" The voice was stern and forceful, yet calm.

Arnvel raised his head but couldn't make out the face before him.

"Mr. Roberts, when I say breathe, I want you to breathe in through your nose. When I say exhale, I want you to breathe through your mouth. Can you do that for me, Mr. Roberts?"

Arnvel nodded that he understood.

"Okay, Mr. Roberts, breathe," the officer instructed.

Arnvel took a short breath and released it immediately.

"Mr. Roberts, don't breathe out till I tell you."

Again, Arnvel nodded his head.

"Mr. Roberts, if we can't get your breathing under control, I will have to call an ambulance. All right, let's try it again."

Arnvel felt a hand cover his.

"Breathe in slowly and hold it."

Arnvel inhaled and held it, focusing more on the voice. *You know how to do this. It's the same technique you were taught in the Army.*

"Now exhale."

Arnvel released his breath. *You can do this.*

"Again, breathe,"

Arnvel took another deep breath.

"Exhale."

Arnvel exhaled. After what seemed an eternity, he was breathing easier. His vision started to clear, and he could see the face that went with the voice. Kneeling in front of him was one of the officers. He looked as if he might be middle-aged. His skin tone was a bit darker than caramel. He was clean-shaven, except for a mustache that reminded Arnvel of Tom Selleck. The top of his head was bald as a monk.

"That's better," the officer said, patting Arnvel's back. "How do you feel?"

The rapid pounding Arnvel felt earlier had slowed almost to normal. "I feel better, thanks to you—" His words were cut short when a patrol car pulled up, and he saw Irene in the back seat. He couldn't get to her fast enough. He wrapped his arms around her and swore he would never take his eyes off her again.

4

~

Chapter Four

In the following months, Arnvel lived in constant fear. Irene was a wanderer and needed 24/7 care. Home health sent out aides—good aides —but she didn't cooperate with them. She would get upset and cry. She would say things like, "I don't know them." or "You don't want to take care of me anymore." or "You don't love me." The aides couldn't do any-thing with her, and her insecurity broke his heart. Eventually, he stopped the home care services. He would do the best he could by himself.

Several falls required visits to the emergency room, but thank God there were no broken bones, only minor injuries. She did, however, have to have stitches one day when she ventured off the front porch without Arnvel knowing it. When she attempted to climb back up the steps, she fell and gashed her head. He had only left her long enough to go to the bathroom, and when he returned, she was sitting on the steps with blood pouring down her face.

He was at his wit's end. He had cried so much since her diagnosis that he didn't know how he could have any tears left. Some nights, he couldn't go to sleep because he was afraid to close his eyes.

Once, he and Irene were sitting in the living room watching TV. He must have dozed off because he was suddenly awakened by knocking at the front door. He noticed Irene was gone. Through the open wooden door, he saw his neighbor Shirley with Irene standing next to her.

Arnvel opened the storm door, and Shirley led Irene inside. "Shirley, what's going on?" he asked, looking from Shirley to Irene. He was scared and confused. "Irene, are you all right? What happened?"

"Settle down," Irene said forcefully, "I went for a walk. Can't I even go for a walk?" She stormed to the bedroom and slammed the door.

Arnvel knew Shirley was a widow and lived a few blocks behind them. Their encounters were always brief but friendly.

Arnvel collapsed on the sofa, physically and mentally drained. What was he to do? He had tried every way he knew to keep her safe. He nodded at Shirley, "Thank you for bringing her home. I hope it wasn't a bother."

"Not at all. That was smart to have her a medical bracelet made," Shirley said as she sat beside him on the sofa. "That's how I knew where she lived." She lightly placed her hand on his. "Mr. Roberts, have you contacted the Department of Human Services? I'm sure they would be happy to help you."

Arnvel was a very proud man. He didn't want to break down in front of Shirley, but there was no holding back the tears that fell. He didn't know how much time had passed, but he could finally take a couple of deep breaths, and his ability to speak returned.

"Of course I have!" he said, pulling his hands away to reach for the handkerchief in his pocket. He dried his face and blew his nose. He squared his shoulders as if he was straightening the weight of the world back on his shoulders. "Aide after aide has come, and she refuses to let them help. She doesn't trust anyone but me."

"Mr. Roberts, it may not be my place, and I know you must love your wife, but I can see the stress you are under. Have you considered putting her in a nursing home? Perhaps there are—"

Arnvel stood posthaste. His eyes hardened and narrowed into slits. His nostrils flared, and through a clenched jaw, he spoke slowly so there was no misunderstanding. "Let me stop you right there, little lady!"

Shirley rose from the sofa and stepped back. She stood there with raised eyebrows, eyes wide, and mouth open.

"How dare you come in here and suggest such a thing! That's my wife 'til death do us part. I think it's best you leave. Thank you for bringing her home, but I can handle it from here. You know where the door is. You can see yourself out."

Shirley got almost to the door when she turned and faced Arnvel again. "Mr. Roberts, I am sorry that I upset you, but I can see that taking care of Mrs. Roberts is taking a toll on you. I know what it feels like. My mother had dementia. I became so overwhelmed that I came very close to a mental breakdown. Eventually, I had to put her in the nursing home, not just for my sake, but for hers as well."

Arnvel struggled to stand a little straighter and met her eyes, "Shirley, that tells me just what kind of daughter you were."

From the stricken look on Shirley's face, Arnvel knew he had gone too far. He watched Shirley leave his home in tears, and he wished he could take his last words back. After some time, he calmed down and started thinking about what Shirley had said. Maybe she had been right. Maybe Irene would be better off in a nursing home.

No! She wouldn't be better off. Sure, we have had a few incidents, but God has blessed us! Everything turned out all right. They could have been worse, but they weren't. He looked up at the wall clock. It read 11:20. He felt confident now that he would be able to sleep. He made sure the front and back doors were locked, and he slipped down the hall to bed.

5

⚬

Chapter Five

Then came the day that would haunt him for the rest of his life. Arnvel awoke to songbirds singing in the magnolia tree outside. Sunshine seeped through the blinds, producing horizontal lines of light on the tan curtains hanging over the window. In the bed beside him, Irene slept and lightly snored. It was almost noon when he looked at the big red digital numbers on his nightstand. *My heavens, I can't believe I slept this late.*

Rushing out of bed, leaving Irene to sleep, he quickly showered. When finished, he went to the kitchen and put on water for coffee. He reached inside the pantry and pulled out a box of Raisin Bran. He put the bowls and spoons on the table. Reaching for the milk from the refrigerator, he heard someone knocking at the front door.

He opened the door where two women waited. One was dressed in a business suit and clutched folders close to her breast. The other wore scrubs. Looking past them, he saw a police car and two officers standing close by. "Yes, can I help you?" Arnvel asked the only thing that came to mind.

"Are you," the woman in the suit started, glancing down at the folder in her arms. "Mr. Roberts, Arnvel Roberts?"

"Yes, ma'am, I am. What can I do for you?"

"Mr. Roberts, I am Olivia Beckett, and this is Judith Dalton." She gestured to a woman wearing scrubs. "I am from the Department of Human Services, and Mrs. Dalton works for Pleasant Hill Nursing Facility. May we come in and talk to you?"

He couldn't say anything at first. Too many thoughts were coming to mind, too many to process. *Maybe they wanted to talk to him about some more services or programs. But what's with the police?* He stepped aside to let them in. "Yeah, come on in."

The ladies stepped across the threshold. Mrs. Beckett looked around as if she was searching for something. "Mr. Roberts, is Mrs. Roberts here?" she asked.

"Yes, but she is still sleeping. Why are the police here? Is something wrong?"

"Mr. Roberts, do you mind if we have a seat? I have some important matters to go over with you, and it might be a bit more comfortable if we sit."

His gut tightened, bile rose in his throat, and silent alarms blared in his head. He hadn't felt a premonition this strong since the Army. Yea, he remembered this feeling. Something terrible was about to happen.

"I think I will stand. Again, I ask you, why are there police outside?"

"Mr. Roberts, it would be better..."

Arnvel interrupted, "No, it would be better if you just spit out what you are doing here, and why are the police involved!"

"Mr. Roberts, we have received some reports that there may be a problem in the home, which has led to Mrs. Roberts having several harmful accidents."

"Hold on, wait a minute." Arnvel waved his hand out as if to stop her words in midair. A wave of dizziness took him, and he crumbled into the sofa's cushions. "You, you think I'm not taking care of her? I, ugh," He closed his eyes and shook his head, "I don't think I understand."

"No. No, Mr. Roberts, we're not saying that at all," Mrs. Beckett quickly stated. "That will be determined by Adult Protective Services after their investigation."

"What investigation!" He struggled to stand but fell back on the couch. Mrs. Beckett reached to try and help him, but he pulled his arm from her grasp. "Don't touch me!" He yelled.

The two police officers entered the living room, not bothering to knock. "Is everything all right here?" one of them asked.

"I don't know if it is or not yet, officer. I'm still at a loss as to what the hell is going on." Arnvel barely had a grip on his temper, but he knew he had to reign it back in. Just then, Irene came in from the hallway.

Sleep was still in Irene's eyes, "Arnvel, you didn't tell me we had company. Is coffee on?"

Arnvel crossed the room and wrapped an arm around her. He escorted her to her favorite chair. For a second, they peered into each other's eyes. Hers were clear, and the spark was back, showing she knew who he was. "They don't want coffee. They're here on business, dear. Sit here, and I'll get your coffee in a bit."

Her eyes landed on the officers. "Why are the police here? Did something happen?"

"We are about to find out," he answered, patting her shoulder. "Aren't we, Mrs. Beckett?"

Arnvel watched as the woman wearing scrubs weaved around, knelt in front of Irene, and took her hand. "I'm Judith, Mrs. Roberts. Glad to meet you."

Irene smiled at the woman, "Glad to meet you, too. Take a seat. Don't kneel like that. It's not good for the knees, you know."

"You are perfectly right." She grabbed an empty chair and pulled it next to Irene. "There, that's better."

"Umm, can we please get back to the reason why all of you are here?" Arnvel snarled. With every fiber in his being, he knew something critical was about to happen.

6

~

Chapter Six

In a professional tone, Mrs. Beckett explained, "Mr. Roberts, I see our visit is upsetting you, but I promise we are only here to help, not only with just your wife but to help you, too."

Arnvel stood beside Irene, his hand resting on her shoulder. He felt his hand shaking, and he hoped she couldn't feel it. As if she could read his thoughts, she reached up and covered his.

"A court order has been issued. Mrs. Roberts is to be put in emergency custody of the state..."

"Whoa, whoa, what the hell do you mean by emergency custody?" Arnvel interrupted. "There is no emergency here, and she isn't going anywhere!"

He felt Irene squeeze his hand, a flash like a warm lightning bolt seared through his hand. He wanted to rip his hand from hers, but he didn't. She turned her head to look at him, and he saw out and out fear. "Where are they wanting to take me, Arnvel?" his wife asked.

"There, there," he said, patting her hand, "they are not taking you anywhere."

"Mr. Roberts don't make this harder than it needs to be," Mrs. Beckett stated firmly. "She will be placed in Pleasant Hill Nursing Facility, and you may visit anytime you like."

Irene wept bitterly, unable to control her emotions. Mrs. Beckett gave the nurse a brief glance and a nod, indicating that she should take his wife away. But the moment the nurse moved, pandemonium broke out.

The nurse stood and took Irene's hand. "Mrs. Roberts, you get to take a ride with me."

Irene continued to cry, but she let the nurse help her up. "But I don't want to go anywhere. I want to stay here."

Mrs. Beckett's eyes softened, "Mrs. Roberts, I'm sorry you and your husband are going through this, but please understand, that we have to make sure you're safe."

"She isn't going anywhere with you or anyone else!" Arnvel wailed, pulling on Irene's arm.

That's when one of the officers came forward and stepped in. "Do you remember me, Mr. Roberts?" He removed his cap to display his bald head.

Arnvel squinted, "Yeah, yeah, I think I do. You helped me the first time my wife was missing." He released Irene's arm.

The officer stepped closer and calmly said, "I didn't get a chance to introduce myself that night, but I'm Officer Graham Matthews."

"Please," Irene sobbed, "don't hurt my husband."

The nurse pulled Irene closer and tried to steer her towards the door. Irene struggled against her. "Everything is going to be all right; they won't hurt him," the nurse said.

"No! I'm not going anywhere without him!" Snot ran from her nose, threatening to reach her mouth.

Arnvel moved toward Irene, but the officer held up his hand, urging him to stay where he was.

"Mr. Roberts, you said I helped you that night. Please, let me help you now. They have a court order to take her. Trust me, Mr. Roberts. Let them do what they need to do. Talk to your attorney, and he will be able to tell you what you need to do next," Officer Matthews said.

"Okay, okay," Arnvel said, bowing his head in surrender, "I trusted you then, and I'm going to trust you now. Can I talk to her before they take her? I might be able to make it a little easier."

"Sure thing," the officer said with a calming smile. "Hold up a minute," he ordered. "Let him have a couple of minutes with her before she goes."

Mrs. Beckett nodded to the nurse, giving her the okay. "Just a couple of minutes. Anything longer will make the separation that much harder."

When the nurse released Irene, she rushed to Arnvel.

He reached and pulled a few tissues from the box on the table. He gently wiped at her nose and then covered her nose. "Blow," he softly said, and she did. "That's my girl." He finished wiping her nose, and without a second thought, he pocketed the dirty tissues.

Arnvel took her hands into his. "Irene, I want you to go with these nice people. I will be right behind you."

"Excuse me, Mr. Roberts," Mrs. Beckett interrupted. Arnvel turned and faced her. The look he gave her made her back up. She squared her shoulders and continued. "It will take some time to get her processed and settled in. It will be best if you wait until tomorrow before you come for a visit. The facility will provide what she needs tonight. You may visit tomorrow and bring her some clothes and personal items if you like."

"Am I going to spend the night somewhere else, Grandpa?" Irene asked in a child-like voice.

Arnvel sighed. She had slipped away. *Maybe that's best.* He returned his attention to his wife, "Yes, but only for a few nights. Just until I get some things straightened out."

"I'll go if you want me to, but only if you promise I get to see you every day, and I don't have to stay longer than a couple of days."

A thin, tight-lipped smile spread across his face, and through slightly clenched teeth, he answered her. "I promise. I will be there every day, and you'll be back home where you belong before you know it."

"Okay, I'll go," she sniffled, "but only because you promised."

"Mrs. Roberts, it's time to go," the nurse informed.

Arnvel kissed her forehead, "I love you. And remember, I'll see you in my dreams.

"I love you too." Irene followed the nurse and was placed in a car.

Arnvel waved to her from the front porch as the car pulled away.

7

~

Chapter Seven

Arnvel had no sleep that dreadful night. He spent long hours going through Irene's things and packing what he thought she might need. He must have packed and unpacked her small suitcase five or six times. Sometime in the early hours of the morning, he made himself stop. He latched the case and rolled it to the front door.

He sat on the front porch drinking coffee. He watched and waited to see if there would be a new dawn. He felt like time had stopped, and life would not go on until Irene was home with him again.

To his sadness, the sun started to rise, spreading its golden fingers across the sky. Sipping his coffee, Arnvel wondered who had called social services. Could it have been her doctor or maybe someone in the emergency room? *"Hell, it could have been anyone."*

He watched the neighborhood come alive, starting their day as usual. "Time waits for no one," he whispered to himself. They waved and yelled good morning. Did they not know his world had crashed down around him?

He couldn't tolerate their happiness any longer. He went back inside. He needed another cup of coffee anyway. He watched the clock and waited for his attorney's office to open.

When the time finally arrived and he called, the secretary told him he would be out of the office for a few days and couldn't be disturbed.

"This is an emergency! I must talk with him now!" He bellowed. He heard the woman gasp on the other end. "Look, I'm sorry. The state has my wife, and I need him to tell me what to do."

"Mr. Roberts, I'm sorry, but all I can do is message him. He will call you when he is available."

He massaged the tight, throbbing muscle in the back of his neck. "I guess I have no choice. Please stress to him that she is alone there and scared. I promised I would bring her home."

"I will, Mr. Roberts," she said with sympathy, "I know this might seem impossible, but please try not to worry. I'm sure everything will work out."

"I don't know about that but thank you.

* * *

The cab pulled up at the nursing home. The driver exited and opened the passenger door for Arnvel. He slowly pulled himself out and paid the driver. The cab pulled away, but he just stood there, looking at the building. He had seen this same building many times before, but now it seemed different somehow, more terrifying.

Its bricks were faded with time, *like the people living inside,* he thought. An old woman with wispy white hair sat outside in a rocking chair. Her head drooped as if she might be asleep, but the chair steadily rocked back and forth.

A nurse or aide appeared from the double glass doors. She doesn't acknowledge Arnvel standing there. Instead, she says something to the woman.

He pulled the handle up on the suitcase, pulled it up the long side-walk, and entered the glass doors the nurse or aide held open for him. "Good morning," she greeted.

"Good morning," he replied as he entered what seemed to be a gathering room. Two women sat on one of the couches, but neither talked. A man who was reading sat in a wing-back chair. Others rolled in their wheelchairs. Arnvel eagerly searched each face, looking for Irene, but didn't spot her.

Finding the offices, he stepped through another glass door. Three women were seated behind desks. One held a phone to her ear. After several moments, the older woman acknowledged him.

"Good morning. What can I do for you?" She smiled as she walked toward him.

"Can you tell me what room Irene Roberts is in, please?" he firmly asked, not returning her smile.

"Are you, her husband?"

"Yes, I'm Arnvel Roberts."

The woman returned to her desk and pecked at her keyboard. "Aww, here she is, Mr. Roberts. She is in room 309. Follow me. These halls can be tricky."

She walked past him, and he fell in behind her, feeling like a child playing follow the leader.

He hated how her heels made that clicking sound with every step she took. *Why on God's green earth don't shoe companies put rubber soles on high-heeled shoes?*

The woman stopped short in front of Arnvel, causing him to stop suddenly to avoid rear-ending her.

"I'm sorry," she tapped her palm to her forehead, "I forgot to introduce myself. I'm Mrs. Holcomb. I'm the administrator here at Pleasant Hill." She offered him her hand.

Holding out his hands, Arnvel said, "Sorry, Arthritis." He didn't want to get friendly with anyone in this place. *What did they expect from him anyway? They did force his wife in here without his permission.*

She sharply inhaled, bringing her hand to her mouth, "Oh, you poor dear! I certainly understand. Well, let me get you to your wife. I know you're anxious to visit."

They continued down the hall, and he followed her to the left. The room numbers were on oversized gold, tarnished plaques— even on the right, odd on the left. Subconsciously, he read off each room number and finally stopped at 309.

"Here we are." The administrator stretched out her arm like a game show model. "If you need anything, just let us know."

"Thank you," he mumbled as he opened the door and closed it behind him.

8

Chapter Eight

There were two beds in the room. The first one was empty. The bed closest to the window had an occupant, but the person's back was to him. He eased closer, careful not to startle whoever lay in the bed. He was sure it was Irene, but he wanted to be positive.

"Irene, are you awake?" he whispered, giving her a little shake.

"Hmm," she moaned.

He removed his hand and stepped back in case it wasn't her.

She moaned again, rolled over, and opened her eyes. When she saw him, she threw off her covers and hurried to his arms. "I knew you would come to take me home."

He was glad to see that she was having a good moment. He broke their embrace and held her at arm's length, carefully looking her over. The only thing he found was a small bruise on her upper left shoulder. "What happened here?" he asked, rubbing the bruise, "Does it hurt? What did they do?"

"It doesn't hurt," she answered as she pulled away from him. "I want to go home!"

She was agitated. She started picking at and smoothing her clothes. He thought it best to try and change the subject. "I brought you some of your things." He smiled as he started to unpack her case. "I know you will be more comfortable wearing your own clothes."

Beside each bed was a three-drawer nightstand. He placed her under-garments and socks in two of the drawers. He started hanging her clothes and gowns in one of the two closets.

He noticed she had calmed down a bit because she was no longer picking at her clothes and was now watching him as he worked. He hung up everything except a navy blue sweatsuit. "Let's get you out of that hospital gown and get you into something better suited."

"Yeah, I don't like my butt showing. I've tried to keep it covered up." Irene laughed.

"Well, we can't have you showing your butt up in here." He laughed with her. "Let's get it covered quick."

He helped her up, removed her gown, and put on her clothes. He sat her back on the bed. "Let's get these things off," he said as he pulled off the hospital socks.

"My feet are going to get cold," she complained.

"No, we're not going to let that happen." He put a pair of her socks on her and slipped on her shoes. "Now, isn't that better? He smiled.

"Yeah, that's better."

There was a gentle *tap* on the door before it opened, and a woman stepped in carrying a tray.

"Good morning, Mrs. Roberts. I've got your breakfast. I hope you're hungry." She placed the tray down on the overbed table. "Do you want to eat in bed or the chair?"

Irene looked at Arnvel. He saw concern covering her face. "Grandpaw, take me home."

Her moment of clarity was gone. He had hoped to spend more time with her as her husband. "You can leave it there. I will see that she eats."

"Won't that be nice, Mrs. Roberts?" The woman said as she gave Irene a mini back rub.

Irene would not look at the woman. She turned her head down and whispered under her breath, "I'll eat when I get home!" Again, she started fidgeting with her clothes.

The woman turned her attention to Arnvel. "You must be Mr. Roberts. I know she is glad to see you. She has been anxious for you to come. I'm Paige. I'm one of the many aides here, and I think Mrs. Roberts is going to be one of my favorites."

"Nice to meet you, Paige," he said as he gently pulled her to the side so Irene couldn't hear what was being said. "I noticed a bruise on her upper arm that she didn't have when she left home. Do you know what happened?"

Paige gently closed the door. "When they brought her in yesterday, she was fine at first. Then she started demanding to go home and wanting to know where her husband was. I and the other aide did what we could to calm her, but her blood pressure spiked, and the nurse had to sedate her. Once the sedative took effect, her blood pressure started to return to normal and she slept through the night. That's why I brought her tray to the room."

Arnvel closed his eyes and shook his head. "I was afraid something like that would happen. Thank you for telling me."

"I know your situation, and I feel for you both. I pray everything works out."

Arnvel felt her words were sincere. They gave him a little more hope. "Thank you for saying that. I will do whatever it takes to get her home again."

"I believe you will, but until then, know that we will take good care of her." Paige opened the door and made her exit.

Arnvel turned from the door, forcing a smile on his face. "All right, little lady, you need to eat before it gets cold."

"I don't want to eat. You said we could go home."

He looked down at her plate because he couldn't look into her eyes. "I have some things to take care of before I can take you home." Still unable to look at her, he cut her stiff scrambled eggs into smaller pieces. "But, as soon as I do," he unwillingly looked at her and smiled the best fake smile he possibly could, "I will sweep you out of here and take you home."

"How long will that take?" She almost shouted.

"I tell you what." He knew he had to change the subject. "If you eat at least a couple of bites, we'll go for a walk. How's that?"

She sighed, irritated. "Ok, but this is stupid!"

He put some egg on the fork and offered her a bite.

She took the bite, chewed once, and spit it out. "That is horrible!"

"Ok, no more eggs." He quickly spread butter and jelly on a piece of toast. "Here you go. Try eating this and drink some of your coffee."

She took the toast from his hand but didn't attempt to take a bite. She dropped her hand to her lap, lowered her head, and cried.

"Oh, Irene." He whispered, taking the toast from her hand. He held her while she cried. She didn't say anything, and neither did he. He wasn't sure how much time had passed, but her crying ceased, and she didn't move or say anything. He thought maybe she had cried herself to sleep. "Irene," He mumbled.

She raised her head and looked at him. A stream of clear slime ran from her nose, down her lips, and dripped from her chin. He reached into his pocket and pulled out his handkerchief. With a tender touch, he cleaned her face.

He had to do something. He wasn't going to wait on the attorney. "Come on, Irene, we're going for a little walk."

Her arm looped through his, and he led her from the room down the hallways. They passed residents who didn't acknowledge them. They seemed to be in their own little world. A nurse or aide hurried toward them. Arnvel's heart raced but slowed when she entered a room with a flashing red light above the door.

They reached the lobby, where two residents sat in chairs looking out a big glass window, and one was reading on the couch. They kept walking. *Please let us get past the office. Please let us get past the office.*

He thought maybe Irene knew what he was trying to do because she kept quiet and looked straight ahead. Where he led, she followed. As they passed the office glass, he glanced to the right without turning his head. He saw one woman at a filing cabinet with her back to them. His next breath came a little easier. They made it to the door. He grinned as he used his forearm to open the door. The door wouldn't open, and an alarm went off. He hadn't noticed the keypad on the left side of the door.

Immediately, Irene covered her ears and used her side to push at the locked door. The woman from the filing cabinet rushed from the office, and a woman in scrubs appeared from a hallway.

"I was only taking her for some fresh air," he said quickly. Of course, he was lying, but he hoped they believed him.

Irene continued trying to push her way through the door, "Let me out. Let me out!" She screamed, as she still covered her ears.

The lady from the office quickly pushed some numbers on the keypad, and the alarm ended. Irene didn't. Arnvel tried to pull her away from the door, but she pulled away and pushed even harder on the door. "Out. I want out!"

The office lady grabbed Irene by the arm, "You're going to hurt yourself, Mrs...." No one saw it coming. Irene turned and slapped the lady from the office across the face. That's when Arnvel recognized that Irene had slapped Mrs. Holcomb, the administrator. Instantly, Mrs. Holcomb released her grip and covered her cheek. Irene returned to pushing on the door.

The woman in scrubs tried to take Irene's hand. "Mrs. Roberts...." Irene started smacking using both hands.

"No, no, no," Irene said each time the woman in scrubs reached for her.

Arnvel was in shock. His wife had never acted like that.

The aide, Paige came up behind and locked both arms around Irene, pinning down her arms.

"Don't hurt her!" Arnvel yelled, finding his voice.

"I promise you, Mr. Roberts, we will not hurt her," Paige reassured him.

"Go and get Kyleigh." Paige directed the woman in scrubs.

"Help. They're hurting me!" Irene cried, struggling against her captor.

"You're hurting her!" Arnvel stepped forward.

Mrs. Holcomb stepped between him and Paige. "She is not hurting your wife, Mr. Roberts. They're merely trying to calm her down. Let them do their job."

"If she gets hurt, I will bring this place down!" Arnvel retorted. His attention was diverted when the other woman in scrubs arrived with a wheelchair and a woman in black scrubs. The one in black scrubs must have been a nurse, Arnvel thought. She pulled a needle from her pocket, pulled its cover off with her teeth, exposed Irene's upper arm with one hand, and submerged the needle with the other.

Within seconds, Arnvel watched Irene's legs turn to wet noodles. The woman pushed the wheelchair closer, locked the brakes, and both women worked together as if they were dance partners. They put Irene into the wheelchair.

"What did you give her?" Arnvel questioned Kyleigh.

"It was no more than a mild sedative. It will keep her calm for a few hours. When it wears off, she should be back to her old self." She touched his arm reassuringly, "I promise, Mr. Roberts. She will be okay. The aides will take her back to her room and put her to bed."

Irene mumbled something, "It's all right, Mrs. Roberts. We're taking you to your room so you can get some rest," Paige explained. "You've had quite the adventure."

Arnvel started to follow as Paige pushed the wheelchair, but Mrs. Holcomb stopped him. "Mr. Roberts, may I talk to you, please?"

"I'll be right behind you, Irene," he called out as the wheelchair continued up the hall. He turned. "This isn't going to take long, is it?" He thought he would get away without a lecture, but he was wrong.

"Just a few moments, please." She opened the door to the office and directed him to enter first, "We can talk in here where it is more comfortable."

9

Chapter Nine

Early the following day, Arnvel sat deep in thought in the back seat of a taxi. The administrator, whose name he couldn't remember, seemed to have believed his story. Well, today was another day, and he had taken some time to make more of a thorough plan.

He pressed the call button on the outside keypad and waited to be buzzed in. He had learned all this during the polite lecture he got yesterday. *For security, an employee must buzz all visitors in and out.* He mocked her word for word in his head. *Only an aide is allowed to take Mrs. Roberts outside.* This infuriated him to no end, but he managed his temper. He didn't want to raise any red flags.

The buzzer sounded, and he entered the door. As he passed the office, he graciously said good morning to the lady who buzzed him in. She smiled and said good morning back to him. He didn't see this one yesterday, so maybe she wouldn't watch him too closely.

When he investigated her room, Irene was not there. *Don't panic. She's here somewhere.* An aide happened to be coming up the hall. "Excuse me," Arnvel said. "Can you tell me where my wife, Mrs. Roberts, is? She's not in her room."

"Sure, she's in the dining room for breakfast." She answered.

"Thank you," he said. He was relieved as he headed to the dining room.

He hadn't paid any attention to the dining room before. There was no need. It was a huge room with lots of windows. A door led to a courtyard, and round tables covered with white tablecloths sat around the room. Residents occupied every table. He finally spotted her at one of the far tables with her back to him. Luckily, the seat beside her was empty.

"Good morning, good morning, beautiful." He kissed her cheek and sat in the empty chair beside her.

"Grandpaw, where have you been? They won't let me go home!"

"Mrs. Roberts, finish eating, and I'll clean you up. Then you can have a nice visit with Mr. Roberts.

Arnvel recognized the aide, but he couldn't remember her name. Thank goodness for name tags. Taking a quick glance, Arnvel said, "Thank you, Paige. That would be nice."

"You're welcome. I've got to take good care of one of my favorite residents, don't I, Mrs. Roberts?" Paige teased while she wiped Irene's mouth. "She's just about finished." The aide glanced at Mr. Roberts.

"I don't want anything else to eat. My grandpaw is here to take me home now. Thank you for taking such good care of me, but I have to get home to take care of my children." Irene's face turned somber, and a single teardrop fell. "I sure do miss them."

Paige dabbed the tear away. "You will see them soon, Mrs. Roberts, and what a glorious day!"

The sudden realization hit Arnvel like a ton of bricks. She was going to die. He didn't know when, but he knew it would come soon. He felt a panic attack coming. He immediately started his breathing technique and managed to get his emotions under control, at least for now.

He took her hand, but she didn't look at him. "I promise you. You will be back with me, and we both shall see our children again."

Irene raised her head, "Arnvel, when did you get here?" She perked up as if she had just seen him, and he guessed in her world she had.

"She has been in and out all morning, but that is to be expected at her stage," Paige whispered.

"I'm ready to go. Let's go," Irene insisted.

"Do you want me to push her for you, or do you have it?" Paige inquired.

"I've got it. I think we'll go sit awhile in the lobby."

"No one has to push me anywhere. I can walk, but they won't let me. They put me in this contraption every time," Irene snapped.

"I guess we will walk to the lobby then," Arnvel laughed.

Paige locked the wheels, helped Irene with the stirrups, and helped her stand. "She has been getting off balance sometimes, so you might want to hold on to her just to be safe. If anything happens, just push the call button around her neck."

"Thank you. I'm sure we will be fine." Arnvel put her arm through his, and they headed to the lobby.

The walk was quiet, and neither talked. When they reached the lobby, it was empty. He knew some residents were still eating. He figured the others went back to their rooms. They sat on the sofa that was closest to the door. He told the taxicab driver to return at 10 a.m. and, if he didn't come straight out, to wait for him and keep the meter running. The driver promised he would.

They sat and talked a bit, but Irene was off in her little world, wherever it might be on the other side of the big picture window. He didn't mind. He could concentrate on his surroundings. He kept track of everyone he saw, where they were, and what they did.

He didn't wear a wristwatch because it flared up his arthritis. He kept checking the time on the big wall clock in the lobby. He has only seen one girl in the office for a while now. *Hopefully, the others are in a meeting and will be till lunch, if I'm lucky.*

When visitors came, Arnvel would watch the woman look up, buzz the visitor in, and immediately return to whatever she was doing without a second look. She had continued this routine all morning. He looked at the clock. It was 9:45.

He waited for the next visitor to walk up the sidewalk to enter the building. His heartbeat was faster, but he took deep breaths. He looked up at the clock. The time was 9:50. When he turned back to the entrance door, he saw three people coming up the sidewalk. They walked slowly because the older woman in the group was using a walker.

Arnvel stood and used his arm to pull Irene to a standing position. "Up we go, Irene. Time to go." He led her to the door.

"Arnvel, are we going home?"

"Shhh, yes. We're going home."

As the visitors approached, he eased Irene to the side, with their backs to the office.

Hopefully, the woman in the office wouldn't recognize them. He watched as the man in the group pushed the keypad, and he heard the buzzer. Arnvel pulled Irene more to the side to make room for the three to enter, making sure their faces were not seen from the office.

The man entered first. "Good morning." He nodded towards Irene and Arnvel as he held the door for the older woman and a younger woman to enter. The man held the door open, and Arnvel and Irene walked through.

Arnvel led Irene down the sidewalk. He dared not to look over his shoulder. They made it as far as the end of the sidewalk when he heard a woman call out, "Mr. Roberts, stop!" He heard running coming up from behind.

Arnvel stopped but didn't turn around. *God, why?*

The woman who came and stood beside them was no other than Mrs. Holcomb. With her was a man that Arnvel had not seen before. He wore a badge that read Stanley, Physical Therapy.

"Mr. Roberts, what do you think you are doing?" Mrs. Holcomb demanded. "Stanley, please help Mrs. Roberts to her room while Mr. Roberts and I talk in my office."

When Stanley reached for Irene, she pulled away from him. "No, we're going home."

Arnvel placed his hand on Irene's shoulder. "It's all right. You go ahead with Stanley, and I'll come to your room when I'm finished with Mrs. Holcomb."

"Okay, but don't take too long. The kids will be waiting on us."

Arnvel hated lying to her. His plan hadn't worked. "We'll be quick, I promise."

Stanley walked Irene up the walk with Mrs. Holcomb and Arnvel following.

Arnvel didn't wait to be asked. He sat in the first chair he came to. He had no strength.

"What were you thinking, Mr. Roberts? Don't tell me you were just taking her out for some air or for a walk.

"I was...."

Mrs. Holcomb held up her hand, "Let me stop you right there. I don't think you understand the severity of your situation, Mr. Roberts. Mrs. Roberts is a ward of the state. Do you know that I could have you arrested for kidnapping?"

"Kidnapping? She is my wife. How can you say kidnapping?"

"I'm not going to call the police, Mr. Roberts. I understand you're hurting. I know you plan to go to court on this situation, but until a decision is made, Pleasant Hill is responsible for your wife's safety and well-being."

Arnvel stood abruptly. He didn't know how he was able to, but he did. "What makes you people think that I can't take care of my wife? I can do everything you do here at this place."

"Mr. Roberts, I'm not going to argue with you. That is between you and the court system. I'm sorry, but I am just doing my job and have rules to follow. Mr. Roberts, I'm sorry to have to do this, but you cannot visit your wife anymore. I have to ban you from Pleasant Hill." Mrs. Holcomb's stern action was more than clear. Arnvel was denied access to his wife.

10

~~

Chapter Ten

* * *

Arnvel suddenly woke up, disoriented. He looked around the room and realized he was in his living room. He must have fallen asleep while he was waiting for Sam. He looked at the wall clock. He still had about fifteen minutes before Sam arrived. He eased himself to the edge of the couch, and with a rocking motion, he slowly stood. He went into the bathroom and splashed cold water on his face. He patted his face and hands dry and stared at his reflection in the mirror.

He looked pale and much older. The usual dark circle under his eyes was darker and puffier. He turned from the mirror in disgust and returned to the living room. He put on a jacket from the closet and picked up the pistol, concealing it in the pocket. He had not handled a gun in many years. He prayed he would not have to use it and that his hands would do the job if he had to.

He took one last look around the house, pulled the awaiting suitcase onto the porch, and locked the front door. He stood and waited for Sam to pull up. He couldn't ask for a better friend than Sam. They had been in the army together and remained friends after. When he told Sam of his plans, Sam didn't hesitate to agree to help. Arnvel promised if he got caught, he would swear Sam was oblivious to what he had planned.

Arnvel saw Sam's car turn onto his street. Pulling the suitcase down one step at a time caused intense pain in his hand. Sam helped him load the suitcase into the trunk, and they pulled away.

"Are...are you sure you want to go through with this?" Sam stuttered. "You could take your chances in court."

Arnvel turned to face Sam abruptly, causing his neck to pop, "Are you saying you don't want to do this?"

"No, I just want to make sure you have weighed all your options before you go too far, and we can't back out."

"I don't have any other options," Arnvel agonized.

"Ok. We're doing this then."

"Yep, we're doing this."

They drove the rest of the way in silence. They pulled up and parked in front of the nursing home, hoping they would not draw any attention to themselves. Perhaps others would think they were doing a drop-off. They had waited till dark, and visiting hours were not over until 9:00.

Arnvel exited the car, readjusting the pistol in his pocket. He pulled the hood up to help hide his face, feeling like he was too old to be wearing a jacket with a hood. But he didn't care. He stood to the side of the door and waited nervously.

He heard the buzz, and the door opened. Arnvel stepped from the side and quickly grabbed the handle. "Oh, I'm sorry. I didn't see you there." The man said politely. "Let me hold the door for you."

"Thank you," Arnvel said in a lowered voice. He stepped into the doorway, sure to keep his head down.

"Have a good night," the man said as the door shut.

Without being noticed, Arnvel made his way to Irene's room. Irene sat in a chair, looking at a blank TV screen. She didn't look at whoever entered her room. He pulled his hood back. "Irene, I'm taking you home."

Irene looked at him with no recognition, "Who are you?"

He moved closer for her to get a better look, "It's me, Irene, Arnvel."

She squinted her eyes, searching his face like looking at the fine print on a contract. "No, you're not my husband. I don't think I know you. I think I'll wait here for him."

Arnvel felt his heartbreak and grief take over. He pushed those emotions aside so he could handle the job at hand. "Arnvel sent me to get you. He is waiting for you at home."

"Oh, well, I'm not dressed to go anywhere."

They had already gotten her ready for bed. "Well, that's ok. Arnvel won't mind if I help you change clothes." He didn't know what else to say to convince her. He just knew they had to hurry before someone came in.

"Oh, no, you won't!" She answered sharply. "If you can pick me out something from that chifforobe over there, I can dress, but you will have to turn your back."

Arnvel picked her out a black sweatsuit and handed it to her.

"Thank you. Now turn around and no peeking. I'm a married woman."

Arnvel turned around and waited for her to dress. Several moments passed, and he heard her grunting a few times. After what felt like an eternity, she told him she was ready.

Looking in the mirror, she smoothed and puffed up her hair. "I should brush my hair."

Quickly, he stepped in, "You look fine. We have to hurry and be as quiet as we can, okay?"

He slowly opened the door and peeked out, checking up and down the halls. Not seeing anyone, he entwined his arm through hers and clutched the pistol in his pocket with his free hand, ready to pull it out at a moment's notice.

They made it as far as the lobby when he heard Kyleigh's recognizable voice. "Visiting hours are over, and you can't take the residents out of the building."

Arnvel turned, pulled out the pistol, and pointed it toward Kyleigh. "This says I can!"

Kyleigh stopped dead in her tracks and threw up her hands. "Mr. Roberts, you don't want to do this."

"Yes, yes, I do. I don't want to hurt anyone, especially you, but I will. I'm taking her out of here. So please, don't try to stop me," Arnvel pleaded.

Paige must have heard the commotion because she appeared in the lobby. When she saw the gun, she stopped just short of Kyleigh. She inched forward. "Mr. Roberts, what are you doing? You know you are not supposed to be here."

Arnvel took his focus off Kyleigh and onto Paige, "Stop right there. Don't come any closer!"

Paige stopped, following suit. She raised her hands. "Okay, calm down. We don't want anyone to get hurt."

Keeping the gun pointed toward Paige, he demanded that she buzz the door open and for Kyleigh to stay right where she was.

Keeping her hands up, Paige slowly inched toward the office. Arnvel stepped backward, closer to the door, pulling Irene with him. "Don't do anything foolish. Remember, I can see you."

Paige reached inside the office and pressed the buzzer.

Using his back, he pushed open the door. "She doesn't belong here either." Arnvel and Irene exited, got into the waiting car, and drove out of sight.

11

༄

Chapter Eleven

Kyleigh immediately called the police. When they arrived, they took an incident report, issued a silver alert, and called out an APB on Arnvel Roberts.

After the police left, Paige and Kyleigh sat at a table in the breakroom. Paige called Mrs. Holcomb while Kyleigh was on the phone with the police. She arrived minutes after the police. She wore blue jeans and a tee shirt, which she would never have worn to work. Her usual tidy hair was thrown up in a ponytail.

Mrs. Holcomb arranged for a nurse and a C.N.A. to arrive early so Paige and Kyleigh could go home. She told them to take the next day off. That was the least she could do. "You girls, go get some coffee or something. Try to relax a little in between call lights. You should be able to go home in about an hour or so."

They both thanked her and went to the breakroom. Kyleigh and Paige cradled their cups of hot coffee. Neither talked, their heads lowered over the steam from their cups.

"What do you think will happen to them?" Kyleigh mumbled, not looking up.

"I'm sorry. I wasn't listening. I was deep in thought. What was the question?" Paige explained.

Paige looked up. "I was thinking out loud. What do you think will happen to them when the police catch them?"

Kyleigh lowered her cup, "Honestly, I'm not sure. I am still trying to get my head wrapped around him coming in here with a gun. I want to think that he wouldn't hurt us, but desperate people do desperate things. I mean, put yourself in his shoes. You could tell how deeply he loves her. There are only two of them. I hate to think what would happen if that were my parents. I believe my dad would do the same thing."

"Yeah. I know my dad wouldn't care if it was my mom. He didn't even bother to get to know me. All I can say is good riddance." Paige waved goodbye in the air. "But that is another story for another time. Mrs. Roberts was one of my favorite patients. Did you know that she lost all three of her children? I don't even want to imagine what something like that would do to a person." Paige agonized.

"Well, I pray we never have to go through that." Kyleigh got up and poured herself another cup of coffee. "Ready for a refill?"

Paige held her cup out. "Sure, fill her up." She took a sip. "Yesterday, while I was dressing Mrs. Roberts, she told me that she used to play the autoharp, and Mr. Roberts played the guitar, banjo, and harmonica. She said they used to go to bars when they were younger, but she called them juke joints. I had to ask her what a juke joint was." Paige laughed. "She said that the bands would call them up to play all the time. They must have been very talented. She told me that Mr. Roberts still picks some when his hands don't hurt, but then he would spend the rest of the day complaining about how much his hands were hurting." Paige laughed again.

"Typical man if you ask me. What is an autoharp?" Kyleigh giggled. "I've never heard of one."

"I had to look it up on the internet myself," Paige admitted. "It looked like a small harp, guitar, and piano combined, played on your lap or a table. Looked complicated, but all musical instruments look that way to me."

Kyleigh listened with her mouth gapped open. "Wow, I'm going to have to look at that."

They both returned to staring into their coffee cups. "You know what?" Paige asked in a lowered voice. "You might think I'm crazy, but I hope they don't find them. I want to be able to imagine them living out their days together."

Mrs. Holcomb entered the breakroom and poured herself a cup of coffee. She propped herself against the counter, "How are you two doing? Is everything okay?"

Kyleigh answered first. "Doing better. Have you heard anything about the Roberts?"

"No, not yet, but I'm sure they will find them. I mean, how far can they get?" Mrs. Holcomb shrugged.

"Mrs. Holcomb, I know you said I could go home, but do you mind if I wait here until you hear something?" Paige pleaded.

Kyleigh quickly stated that she felt the same.

"Are you two sure you want to do that? Haven't you two been through enough already?" Mrs. Holcomb asked.

Paige and Kyleigh glanced at each other and then at Mrs. Holcomb. In unison, they answered. "We're sure."

"If that's what you want to do." Mrs. Holcomb headed to exit. "Oh, by the way, your relief is here, so clock out, and I'll let you know when I hear anything. You two must have gotten close to Mrs. Roberts these past few days. I suspect you know that is not a good idea in our line of work."

Mrs. Holcomb left the break room, and Kyleigh and Paige stared at each other, not believing what their boss said.

"It's easy for her to say that. She doesn't spend time with the patients as we do," Paige stated.

Kyleigh got up and picked up the almost empty coffee pot. She poured what was left down the sink. "I envy CNAs sometimes. You get to know the patients more in-depth than nurses do. It's more charting and paperwork for us, and the state has added more on top of that." She put in a fresh filter with coffee and started the coffee pot before she returned to her chair.

Paige covered Kyleigh's hand with hers, "That may be true, but that doesn't mean you can't have empathy and compassion for your patients,"

Kyleigh leaned closer to Paige and whispered, "I hope they get away too."

12

~

Chapter Twelve

* * *

Sam pulled in front of the Gray Hound bus station. "Are you sure you don't want me to wait with you?"

Arnvel got out on his side and went to the driver's window. Sam rolled down his window, "This is where we part ways, dear friend. You have done enough. Remember our story. You didn't know anything about what I was going to do." He got Irene from the car and closed the door, "Thank you, Sam."

Sam covered his friend's hand, "Don't get caught."

Arnvel and Irene entered the bus station. Arnvel led Irene to one of the seats closest to the ticket purchase windows. "Irene, I need you to sit right here. I will be right back." He tried to pull away, but she wouldn't let him.

She had not spoken since they left the nursing home. "Arnvel, please don't leave me again."

When she said his name and looked into her eyes, he knew she was alert and in the moment. "I promise. I won't leave. We're going home, back where we need to be." He kissed her forehead before he went to the ticket purchase window.

He pulled cash from his pants pocket and held it in his hands. He had gone earlier to the bank and withdrawn everything they had from their checking account, closing the account. The man in the barred enclosure looked at him. "Can I help you, sir?"

Arnvel kept his head down as much as possible, "Yes, I need two one-way tickets to Jacksonville Beach, Florida, please.

The man typed on his computer, "There will be a brief delay in Atlanta, Georgia, to pick up passengers, but other than that, it is a straight-through."

Arnvel unrolled the cash in his hand, "That's fine. How much?"

The man gave him an amount, and Arnvel gave him the money. The man printed out the tickets and handed them to Arnvel with his change. "The bus should arrive by 11:15 and should be on time."

Arnvel lifted his eyes to the huge clock that hung behind the clerk. Over two hours to wait for the bus. He took the tickets and his change, "Thank you." He returned to Irene and took the seat beside her. "It won't be long now." He held her hand and said a silent prayer.

"You're taking me home, right? No more of that place?" She squeezed his hand, not realizing the pain she was causing.

"Not if I can help it. I will do everything in my power to be with you. I hope you know that, Irene." He pulled her entangled hand from his and laid her hand on top instead. He looked around the bus station. He counted ten people waiting for a bus, not including himself and Irene. This must be a slow night. They were spread out as if everyone wanted to keep their distance from the others. Perhaps everyone had a secret or was running away from something. A security guard sat at his little station, a pistol holstered at his side. He spotted a vending machine on the far wall, and his stomach reminded him he had not eaten since this morning. "I'm hungry, are you? I haven't eaten yet. I'm famished."

Irene picked imaginary fuzz from her sweatshirt. "I want an RC if they have it. They wouldn't let me have soda." She didn't look up.

Arnvel fed money into the machine and got two RCs and a pack of cheese crackers. He carried the sodas in the crook of his arm. When he passed the trash can, he stopped and glanced around to make sure no one was looking. Nonchalantly, he pulled the pistol from his pocket and buried it under the trash.

While he ate his crackers, he watched the entrance for police and watched the clock on the wall. The last time he checked the clock, it read 10:45 pm. Irene had finished her RC and had fallen asleep with her head on his shoulder. A young couple had come in and seated themselves in the seats across from them. The young woman smiled at him, and he smiled back, hoping she didn't want to strike up a conversation.

He was so tired. He couldn't remember ever being this tired, physically and emotionally. He didn't remember closing his eyes, but he must have. Somewhere in a far-off distance, someone was calling his name. "Mr. Roberts, Mr. Roberts, we need you to wake up now."

Arnvel slowly opened his eyes, and two policemen stood over him and Irene with their hands on their holstered firearms. He recognized one of the officers as the one who helped him with his panic attack the first time Irene had gone missing. He was the first to speak. "Mr. Roberts, we don't want any trouble here, but you must come with us.

Arnvel looked at the clock on the wall. This time, it read 11:05. If only his luck had held out for another ten to fifteen minutes, they would have been on their way.

Irene stirred and lifted her head from Arnvel's shoulder. "Are you two going to Florida. too?" she asked. "We're going to go swimming, aren't we Grandpaw?"

Arnvel didn't look away from the officers. "I think we will have to put our trip off for a while. Isn't that right, Officer Graham Matthews?" Irene didn't say anything. She lowered her head, picked at the imaginary fuss on her clothes, and tossed it onto the floor.

Officer Matthews grinned. "I'm glad you remember me. This is my partner, Timmons. You got yourself in quite a situation here, Mr. Roberts."

Arnvel moaned as he stood. "Yeah, I guess I did, but I had to do what I had to do. Just like you have to do what you have to do."

Timmons unhooked his handcuffs. Matthews waved for him to put them away. "There will be no need for those, right, Mr. Roberts?"

Arnvel shook his head, "No, you won't need those. I won't cause a scene."

Matthews took a step closer to Arnvel. "I'm glad to hear that. Mr. Roberts, do you have any weapons on you that we need to know about before we search you?"

Arnvel lowered his eyes and again shook his head, "No, I don't have anything on me. The gun is in that trash can over there." He motioned toward the trash can.

Matthews gestured to Timmons to check for the gun. He put on a pair of blue gloves, rummaged through the garbage, and pulled up the pistol. He nodded to Matthews as he slid the gun into an evidence bag.

Matthews patted Arnvel down. Arnvel could feel everyone staring at him. The young woman who had smiled at him earlier now stared at him with a puzzled look. She was not smiling now. Irene didn't say anything. She watched Matthews search her husband.

Matthews grabbed a vacant chair and set it opposite Arnvel. "Take a seat, Mr. Roberts." Several signs clearly said, **Do Not Move Chairs!** But Arnvel knew no one would say anything to the officers about it.

"Now, here's what has to happen. Officer Timmons will take Mrs. Roberts back to the nursing home, and you and I are going down to the station. I will let them leave first so she doesn't have to watch you being put in a squad car. I want to accomplish this without a big ruckus, and I'm sure you don't want that either."

Arnvel's eyes teared up, and he brushed them away. *I'll have plenty of time to cry later.* "I understand, but can I talk to her and say goodbye?"

Irene suddenly raised her head in Arnvel's direction, "Goodbye. Where are you going, Grandpaw?" she asked.

Arnvel didn't know how to say goodbye without breaking down, but he knew he had to. He knew this would be the last time he would see her. He didn't care that he was going to jail. Without her, everywhere was going to be hell for him.

He cupped her face, "You are going to get to ride in the police car. You have long wanted to do that and now is your chance. What do you think about that?"

Irene stood, her face lit up and smiling. Then her expression turned to worry.

"Don't worry about me, Irene, I'll be fine. I will always be right here." He took her hand and placed it over her heart. "You will be right here." He said as he placed her hand over his heart.

As he spoke, Arnvel saw an awareness in her that he had not seen in a long time. She was the Irene he had fallen in love with and married. Was she comforting him, or was he seeing what he wanted to see?

She stood on her tiptoes and kissed him softly on the lips. "I'll see you in my dreams." She turned toward Officer Timmons, "I'm ready for my ride now," she said in a child-like voice. Her awareness was now gone.

As the officer led the excited Irene to the door, Arnvel broke from his trance-like state, "Irene," he yelled.

She stopped and turned to face him.

"I'll come for you when the time comes. Until then, I'll see you in my dreams." The tears came, but he had a smile on his face. He stood there with Officer Matthews and watched Officer Timmons help Irene into the back seat and buckle her in, and then he watched them drive away. He faced Officer Matthews, "I'm ready now."

13

ᙯᙯ

Chapter Thirteen

Mrs. Holcomb entered the breakroom where Paige and Kyleigh sat, awaiting news about Mrs. Roberts. Both had their heads laid on the table as if they were small children in school.

"They found them!" Mrs. Holcomb burst.

Both heads raised quickly. "Are they all right?" Paige blurted out. "Where did they find them?"

"At the bus station, and they are all right, thank God," Mrs. Holcomb answered.

"What..." Kyleigh hesitated. "What will happen to Mr. Roberts? Will they put him in jail?"

Mrs. Holcomb looked at Kyleigh, puzzled, "Well, I'm not sure. I guess the courts will decide. Why do you ask?"

Kyleigh fidgeted with her coffee cup. "I was just curious, that's all."

Mrs. Holcomb's eyes narrowed, "You have to remember, he kidnapped Mrs. Roberts by gunpoint. That's serious."

"I know, but no one was hurt," Kyleigh said.

"Well, anyway," Mrs. Holcomb squared her shoulders, "they are bringing her back here. They're on their way. I thought you two would want to know."

Paige threw her head back, "Can we see her when she gets here, just to make sure she's ok?"

"Sure, but don't stay too long. She has been through enough and needs to rest, and so do you two."

Paige crossed her heart, "We promise. We won't stay too long, and we'll go home right after."

"I'm going to hold you to it, understand?"

Kyleigh stood, picking up her cup. "Sure thing, Mrs. Holcomb." She picked up Paige's cup, and placed it in the sink with hers. "Do you want to go wait in the lobby?"

"Sounds like a plan. Let's go," Paige answered.

The hallways were empty and quiet. When they rounded the corner, an older woman was behind the nurse's station. "Kyleigh, Paige, why are you two still here? We thought y'all went home, considering what happened. Are y'all ok?"

Kyleigh crossed her arms and leaned across the counter, "Thank you, Carol, for coming in early to relieve me. But we're okay. We were waiting for news about Mrs. Roberts. I guess you know she is on her way back?"

"Yes. Mrs. Holcomb told me and Lora."

"Where is Lora? We haven't seen her," Paige asked.

Carol returned a chart to the cart. "She's with Mr. Stanfield. He's having a rough night."

"Another one? His insomnia is becoming more frequent. We should inform the doctor," Kyleigh stated. "He is wearing us out."

"*Whew!*" Lora breathed, "I think he's down for the count." Lora rested her head on her crossed arms on the counter. "I thought you guys went home?"

"We decided to..." Paige was interrupted by the door buzzer.

They raced to the lobby just in time to see a police officer and Mrs. Roberts walk in the door. Paige grabbed a wheelchair that was used for emergencies.

"Welcome back, Mrs. Roberts. I'm so happy you're all right," Mrs. Holcomb said, placing her hand on Irene's back.

Irene shrugged her hand off and stumbled. Hands quickly reached out. Paige won the draw and eased Irene into the wheelchair.

"I'm not all right. This man," Irene pointed her finger at the police officer. "He won't take me back to the bus station. We're going to Florida."

The officer started to say something, but Mrs. Holcomb stepped in. "Thank you, officer, for returning her, but we have it from here. I'll buzz you out." Mrs. Holcomb reached inside the office door and pushed the buzzer.

"Hey there, pretty girl. Will you take me back to the bus station?" Irene looked up at Paige.

Paige knelt so she could be at Irene's eye level. "I'll tell you what. Why don't I get you cleaned up first?"

"But I'll miss the bus," Irene pleaded.

Paige covered Irene's hand. "If you miss the bus, you can catch the next one."

Irene leaned in closer to Paige. "You promise?"

"I promise."

Paige started to push Irene to her room, but Mrs. Holcomb stopped her. "Paige, let Lora take her. You're not clocked in, and corporate will be here in a few hours.

"No, I want her to take me," Irene insisted, nodding toward Paige.

Mr. Stanfield walked towards the lobby, "Hey, I can't sleep."

"Lora, you take care of Mr. Stanfield," Mrs. Holcomb barked. "Paige, you can take Mrs. Roberts, but clock in."

Lora left to take Mr. Stanfield back to his room before he could wake anyone. Paige started once more to Irene's room when Kyleigh stopped her. "Can I go with Paige?"

"Yes, go on." Mrs. Holcomb waved her on. "Go ahead and clock in. too."

"I'm going to get Mrs. Roberts her meds and something to help her sleep," Carol headed off down the hall.

Kyleigh put Irene on her bed while Paige got the wash pan ready.

"I know she's not going to take me to the bus station, but that's okay," Irene said.

Kyleigh took her hand, "Why do you say that?"

"Arnvel told me he would come for me when the time comes, and I'm all right with that."

14

∽

Chapter Fourteen

Arnvel watched Matthews in the rearview mirror, and then their eyes met. Arnvel remained silent.

"Mr. Roberts, I can only imagine what you and your wife are going through, but I want you to know, I feel empathy for you both. I will stay with you while you are being processed. I am praying that will make it a little easier for you.

As promised, Matthew escorted Arnvel through the police station and stayed through the booking process. He even asked to be the one to escort Arnvel to lockup. He unlocked the cell door and let Arnvel step through. "Mr. Roberts, you will be in my prayers," the officer said as he closed the door. The sound of the lock echoed off the stone walls.

Using the bed's metal frame, Arnvel eased down onto the bare mattress. His pain sparked, and he knew there would be no pain medication for him tonight. Maybe he deserved that. He rested his head on the pillow and prayed for a swift ending.

He awoke to the clanking of metal and someone calling out. "Rise and shine, Mr. Roberts." Opening his eyes, he saw he was within the same walls and wearing the same state-issued clothes he had fallen asleep in. The guard held out Arnvel's clothes and some toiletries, "It's time for your bail hearing. Wash up and change." The officer left without saying another word.

Arnvel was led through the door to the courtroom. A few steps in, he saw a small closed-off section where three other men were seated. The guard told him to take an empty seat, and Arnvel did what he was told. He knew he should be thinking about his situation, but he could only think about Irene and the agony in his hands. He tried massaging one after the other, but that only made matters worse. *"Hurry up and get this over with. Lock me up, throw away the key, I don't care. I need this pain to stop!"*

"All rise!"

Arnvel was snatched back to the moment. He stood, using the railing for support.

"Be seated!"

Still using the railing, he eased back down. The first man was called up for armed robbery. The bail was set at $25,000. The second man was called. He was charged with drug possession with intent to distribute. This was his third offense. His bail was set at $10,500.

"Arnvel Roberts!" the bailiff called.

He stood, using the railing and whatever was in reach to steady himself, he walked to the podium where the public defender waited for him. "Mr. Roberts, just let me do the talking for you, and I might just get you out of here by tonight."

"Your Honor, Mr. Roberts..."

The judge shook her head and waved her hand. "No need for all that Bradley. There will not be any bail set in this case."

Arnvel's knees weakened, and his head dropped. *Do whatever you want. I just don't care anymore.*

"But your Honor..." Again, she shut the public defender down.

The judge's features softened, "Mr. Roberts, what do you have to say for yourself?"

He raised his head and locked eyes with the judge. "Your Honor, I am an old man who had the love of my life taken away and forced into a nursing home. If you're asking me if I'm guilty of taking my wife from the nursing home so we can finish our lives together, then Judge, I'm guilty. If given the chance, I would do it again."

"Well, Mr. Roberts, I can tell you this. I feel for you and your wife, and if you would have given the system a chance and the time, things might have worked out differently for you both."

This time, Arnvel shut her down, "You Honor, that's the problem. We don't have that time."

She broke their eye contact and shuffled her papers, "Mr. Roberts, my heart goes out to you, but what you did was wrong. You could be sentenced to a lengthy prison sentence. Because of your age and the situation, you will be admitted to the V.A. hospital and undergo a psychiatric evaluation. Your sentence will follow their recommendations. I wish you the best, Mr. Roberts. You are dismissed.

* * *

For days, Arnvel endured the tests and the questions. So many questions. He felt like a shell of a man. Nothing existed within him but guilt and shame. When he stood before the judge a second time, he was told that he should remain in the care of the State Veterans Nursing Home. He was not surprised.

He settled into the V.A. nursing home. He ate what he could keep down and slept when he could keep the dreams at bay.

* * *

Irene's illness had progressed. Most days, she lived inside her mind. Her words were limited at times. Sometimes, she would speak plain as day, but other days, she would struggle to pronounce a single word. She lost her ability to walk and feed herself. She had to be coerced into taking her medications and tending to her daily personal hygiene. "Kids came today."

Paige slowed the brushing but didn't stop, "That sounds nice. I hope you had a good visit."

Irene turned her head to see Paige "Yes, but strange."

"How was it strange, Mrs. Roberts?"

"They grew up fast. They had to tell me something."

The other times Irene said anything about seeing her children, she referred to them as small children. Another decline in Irene's illness became obvious. She would have to let Kyleigh know so she could document the change on Irene's chart. "They do grow up fast. What did they have to tell you?"

Irene smiled, "Arnvel will be here soon to take me home."

Paige stopped brushing Irene's hair and shivered. "I bet you are ready for a good night's sleep after your visit today. I'll tuck you in."

Irene didn't argue. She let Paige wheel her to the bed and help her in.

* * *

When the rays of sunshine hit Arnvel's eyes, he didn't open them. He pulled the covers up over his head. He played memories of Irene and him through his mind. They were playing on a stage somewhere. He was on the banjo, and she had her autoharp. They danced to *Faded Love,* close and staring into each other's soul. He remembered his kids burying him in the sand on the beach as Irene watched and laughed at their silliness. He didn't know when the reminiscing stopped. Arnvel died later that morning.

* * *

Paige filled Kyleigh in about the change in Irene. "I don't know how to explain it, but something has changed with her. I can't shake the feeling that something is about to happen."

"We knew this would happen, Paige. All we can do is to be there for her and make her as comfortable as possible. Let me finish this, and we will go look in on her.

Kyleigh rushed to finish her charting. Paige's report concerned her. They entered the room together. As they approached Irene's bed, they saw she was awake. Her eyes were glazed over, and she stared at the wall across the room.

Paige sat on the bed beside her and took her hand, "Why are you not asleep? I thought you were calling it a night?"

Irene didn't answer. Her focus was still on the wall.

Kyleigh pulled the blood pressure monitor from her pocket, wrapped it around Irene's arm, and squeezed the bulb. She watched the needle and listened to the heartbeats. She shook her head at Paige.

Paige's head dropped.

"He's here," Irene whispered. Her eyes were mere slits focused on the blank wall.

"Who's here, Mrs. Roberts?" Kyleigh questioned, kneeling on the floor.

"H-h-h-he's he-e-re-," Irene had trouble forming her words, which came slowly. "Take... me... home."

Paige and Kyleigh looked at each other, both crying silent tears.

Paige traced imaginary lines across Irene's forehead. "Go with him, Irene. Let him take you home."

Paige and Kyleigh stood starkly still, mouths gaped, and eyes fixed on the dear woman. Irene reached out her hand and whispered in a hushed voice. "Thank you," and Irene's eyes closed into eternal sleep.

15

***

Epilogue

Arnvel felt himself being pulled from his body. He found himself standing in a room across from Irene. He didn't know if she could see or hear him. Her eyes were half opened. Even with the covers, her body looked thin, and her face was pale. He called to her in a soft voice. "Irene." She didn't stir.

Again, he called, "Irene." This time, he knew she heard him. She moved her head slightly. He felt her eyes on him. She displayed the tiniest of smiles. Then it was gone.

He watched as Kyleigh and Paige entered. Their distress filled the room. It pleased his ears when Irene said, "He's here." His heart overflowed with joy.

Arnvel didn't think the girls would believe Irene that he was there and going to take her home. Blessed tears fell when Paige told her to go with him. He reached his hand out towards her, and she reached for his.

They walked hand in hand among the clouds, talking and laughing. When they reached the pearly gates of Heaven, Peter stood awaiting their arrival. He motioned the gates to open, and they opened wide. Peter motioned for them to enter. "Welcome home."

Enjoy this free gift. A poem that partners with this story.

Life Faded not the Love
Previously Published in
"Kisses from the Mind to the Soul"

They danced to Faded Love and held onto each other tight
Their whole lives ahead of them with nothing but the moment in their
sight
Years came and went just like the problems that arose
More years came and with it the effects of age
The state came and forced them apart and suddenly began to change
He was told he could not see her and taking her home could not be done
He was not going to accept that and returned home to get his gun
With the influence of the gum, into the night they fled
Together again, the tears of joy were shed
When the police found them, again they were torn apart
As they were separated, he promised they would be together again just
like in the start
Time later the couple passed away, each one was alone and each with a
broken heart
God reunited them, and they will never again be a part

16

〰

Authors Note

To my Wonderful Readers,

This story is a homage to a love that battled pain and hardship. I want to treasure and pass on this legacy to my family and descendants. The following pages display the newspaper articles that narrated this incredible story and I have added the photos I found on my investigation for this story

17

~

Newspaper Articles

For the love of his wife

Man's heartbreak leads to incident

· THE CHARLOTTE OBSERVER Tuesday, July 27, 1993 · 3C

By GARY WIREMAN *The Gaston Observer*
Staff Writer

GASTONIA — Relatives knew David Roberts was devastated that his wife of 50 years had been placed in a nursing home, but they never thought it would come to this:

Saturday night, Roberts, 71, walked into South Haven Long Term Care, clutching a .25-caliber pistol, and ordered nurses to fetch 78-year-old Irene Roberts, police say.

He escorted his wife to a waiting car, driven by a friend who was unaware of what David Roberts was doing, police say.

Officers found the couple several hours later, sitting in the Charlotte bus station, confused but unharmed.

On Sunday, Irene Roberts, who suffers from the brain disorder Alzheimer's disease, was back at South Haven.

Her husband — a disabled veteran who relatives say has long-standing health problems of his own — was at the VA hospital in Salisbury, undergoing psychiatric observation.

It's unclear whether charges will be filed.

"He just wanted her back," said Roberts' brother, Joel Roberts of Gastonia. "But he can't even care for himself."

Childless, the Robertses moved to Gaston County several years ago from Florida, where they had lived for 40 years, Joel Roberts said.

David Roberts and his wife stayed with Joel Roberts for several months before moving to an apartment in Dallas.

Over time, health problems worsened, Joel Roberts said.

Irene Roberts grew more disoriented, more dependent on her husband. David Roberts was unable to help. Neighbors eventually called the Gaston County Department of Social Services.

Several months ago, the DSS took custody of Irene Roberts and placed her in South Haven on Marietta Street.

David Roberts was barred after he recently tried unsuccessfully to escort his wife from the home using a taxi, Joel Roberts said.

His brother was becoming more desperate, Joel Roberts said.

"He was going to call the congressmen, and he was going to call the attorney and all that sort of stuff," Joel Roberts said.

"Apparently, he took matters into his own hands."

THE CHARLOTTE OBSERVER Tuesday, July 27, 1993 3C

His love led him to take wife from rest home

By JOE DePRIEST
Staff Writer

GASTONIA — The newlyweds once danced their nights away to swing tunes like "Faded Love."

Fifty years later when they were elderly and sick and forced to live apart, the old song rekindled their passion.

Relatives say bonds between David and Irene Roberts still run deep. So deep, that on Saturday David Roberts brought a gun to a Gastonia rest home and took his wife, police said.

"His love for his wife hasn't faded," said David Roberts' brother, Joel Roberts of Gastonia. "He wanted his wife back. He'll do it again if he gets half a chance."

David Roberts, 73, a disabled veteran, entered the South Haven Long Term Care building on South Marietta Street, Saturday around 7 p.m. and said he wanted to remove his 76-year-old wife, police said.

She suffers from the brain disorder Alzheimer's disease.

"The nurse told him, 'Why, you know you can't do that,'" said South Haven supervisor Joyce Bivnet on Monday. "Then he told her, 'This says I can' and pointed a gun."

Police said Roberts escorted his wife to a waiting car. A friend who was unaware of what was happening was the driver.

Several hours later officers found the couple sitting in the Charlotte bus station.

They had been to Jacksonville Beach, Fla., where they'd tried to elope 49 years before moving to Gastonia a few years ago.

Authorities have placed Irene Roberts in an undisclosed rest home while David Roberts is undergoing psychiatric observation at the VA Medical Center in Salisbury.

Relatives said both David and Irene Roberts had health problems that worsened over the years.

Several months ago, neighbors notified the Gaston County Department of Social Services. DSS investigated and got a court order to place her in South Haven. It's unclear where he was living.

Neighbors sent a stream of letters. Roberts requested the couple not be placed together. DSS wouldn't comment on the case.

David Roberts' sister, Elsie Roberts, 69, of Dallas, N.C., thinks the couple never oppose the separation.

"They're growing for each other," she said. "They won't live long apart. They've always been in love. What I can't see is what God put together, let no man put asunder."

Relatives said the couple had their problems and that David Roberts sometimes drank too much.

But they said love always overcame the troubled times.

"Whichever way the wind blew, they stuck together," Elsie Roberts said.

She remembers them dancing close together in their younger days to the western swing of Texas-born fiddler Bob Wills.

The Roberts always considered "Faded Love" their song.

"He first saw me, I held on," Elsie Roberts said. "And it still expresses the way they feel."

18

❧

Photos

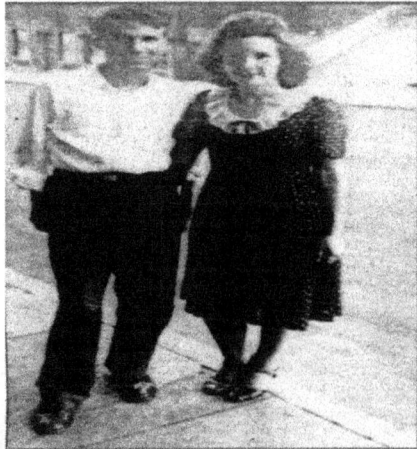

Arnvel and Irene after they were married

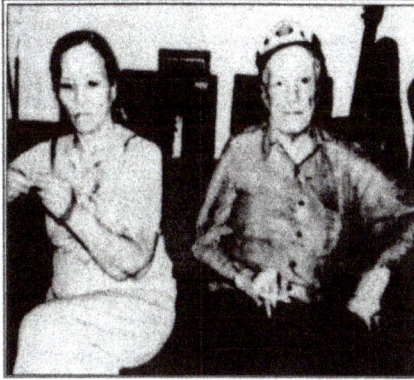

Last known photo taken together

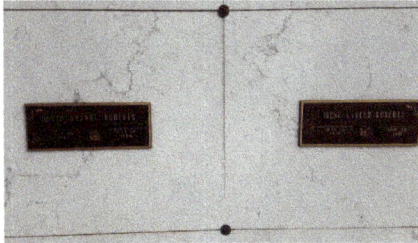

Burial Site at Gaston Memorial Park in
Gastonia, North Carolina

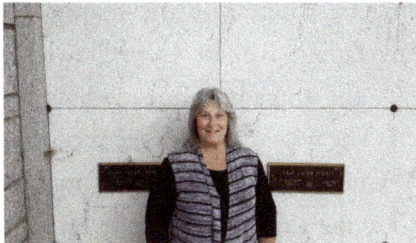

Me at their burial site

Afterword

The question lingers: where was the family during those pivotal moments? When my father, Robert Guy Crawley, passed away from tuberculosis in 1979, the threads connecting us to our grandparents frayed and unraveled. The why remains a silent echo across the years. My dad's brother Larry Crawley, and sister, Jo Ann Marvin, departed this world prematurely, leaving gaps in the family tapestry. However, I have managed to get in touch with some remote cousins on my father's side of the family, through Facebook.

In those days, I called Arkansas home. My mother and siblings resided in North Carolina, unaware of our grandparents' whereabouts until the newspaper's ink etched their story into public circulation. When my mom, Julie, and siblings, Wanda and Karen visited the nursing home, my grandmother revealed selective recognition. My brother, Robert, was her Bobby, a cherished memory of our dad, etched in her heart.

Yet, the veil over the orchestrators of separation remains unlifted. Perhaps they guard their reasons, hidden away like precious relics.

My grandparent's saga, woven with threads of loss and longing, resonates across time. May it inspire resilience and compassion on your journey.

Thank you for reading and I hope the story touched you as it has me.

S.R. Crawley, AKA Sherri Crawley-Phelps-Croom

19

〜

Also by Sherri Croom

S.R. Crawley explores a diverse range of genres, refusing to confine her writing to a single category. If you appreciate variety, she is the perfect author for you.

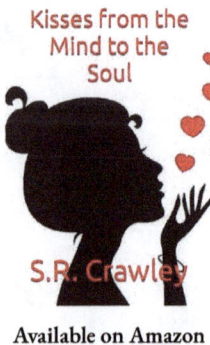

Kisses from the Mind to the Soul

S.R. Crawley

Available on Amazon

Many of the poems you will read in this book are based on events in the author's life. Some will tug at your heart strings and others may make you stop and think... Some of the poems however; are from the authors most darker regions. S. R. Crawley proves to have different personalities when it comes to writing poetry. Take a journey with S.R. Crawley as she blows Kisses from her Mind to your Soul.

Michelle, Eugene, and Billy are strangers. But they share a bizarre and fatal coincidence. They all dropped a shoe on a highway and met their doom. Three stories reveal how they lost their shoe and how a girl in a blue wagon connects them.

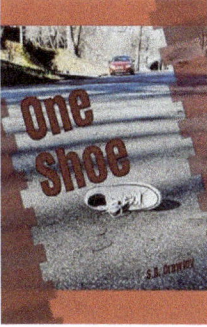

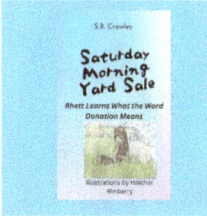

Available on Amazon

Rhett is excited about helping his mom with the yard sale. That is until a little girl picks up and wants her mother to buy his favorite teddy bear, Teddy.

He learns that the little girl lost her teddy bear in a house fire. What is he to do?

Available on Amazon

Your child will learn along with Rhett about the Christian principles of compassion and generosity.

Enjoy this keepsake book that includes coloring pages for your child and a short Bible study where your child, or you, can write what he/she has learned.

Would be a great learning tool for a Sunday School lesson. Bible verses are from the International Children's Bible version.

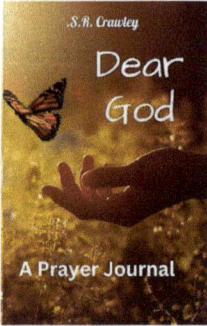

Available on Amazon

A prayer journal is a powerful tool for spiritual growth, self-awareness, and building a deeper connection with God. Start today, and let your written prayers become a testimony of His grace and guidance.